ULTIMATE JUICING RECIPES
For Healthy Living

I0413820

ROY NOLAN

PAVO
PRESS

of the use of information contained within this document, including, but not limited to, —errors, omissions, or inaccuracies.

Trademarks:

PAVO Press and the PAVO Press logo are trademarks or registered trademarks that may not be used without written permission. All other trademarks are the property of their respective owners. PAVO Press is not associated with any product or vendor mentioned in this book.

FIRST EDITION

ISBN-13: 978-1-5427-0751-0
ISBN-10: 1-5427-0751-X

Copy Editor: Tom Edwards
Cover Designer: Annie Eaves
Nutrition Analysis: Sharon Tafoya

To friendship and my readers,

who make my world more meaningful

CONTENTS

Wait!!
Before you continue...
Would you like to read more
of such books for FREE?

For a Limited Time Only!
We will be giving away
Free Membership exclusive
to the first 50 subscribers.

The link will be available at the end of the book. As our member, you will be receiving *LIFETIME Updates* on all our latest promotions, upcoming new books and new book releases, and free books or gifts that we occasionally pamper our loyal members. If you have benefited from our book and find our book useful to you, please remember to leave a **positive review** for us on Amazon. It will motivate us to produce better quality books for your reading pleasure and needs.

THANK YOU!

Chapter 1

Introduction

Do you want to lose weight? Are you getting a hard time to have a healthy lifestyle? No time to prepare for a healthy breakfast because you're late? Worry no more, for this book will surely help you. Inside this book are 50 real juicing recipes that are not only healthy, but deliciously healthy, that will help you throughout your day. Juicing is not only for breakfast. It can be anytime you want. It can be before you hit the gym, or before you sleep. So, this means, that you can be healthy all day!

It is handy, and requires no long time to prepare. All you have to do, is prepare it for not more than 15 minutes, and you can drink it wherever you will go. So, time will not be a reason why you can't be healthy.

Why spend money on expensive juices where you're not sure if they are naturally healthy, when you, yourself, can do it on your own. If you'll reason out that you don't how, then this book is perfectly right for you! Written inside this book are natural ingredients, like fruits and vegetables, and easy to understand instructions to help you what to do. These recipes' ingredients are well researched to combine the right fruits and vegetables to complement each other's taste, and have the desired healthy juice that you need. We also have written the nutritional information, so that you will be guided on what vitamins you have got, and its benefits.

Choose the juice that you don't only need, but the juice that you would like.

Chapter 2

The Power in Real Juicing: How healthy is it?

We have so many things that we want to do in this life. We want to travel the world, get married and have children. But we can't do all these things if our body is not in condition, right? How can we travel, how can we do all these things if our body is sick, lying in the hospital? No one can do the things that we want but ourselves. That is why living a healthy lifestyle and getting the right vitamins that our body needs, is a must.

Fruits and vegetables are one of the best sources of vitamins, minerals, and other nutrients that we need to perform our very best in our everyday life. But what if you don't eat veggies? Because veggies are not so likable, and you hate it because of distasteful taste. Will it be the end of your healthy self? No! Of course, not! Because that is when real juicing comes. Veggies when juiced and combined with the right fruit or another vegetable, it can be magical, you won't expect its outcome, it can be a delicious tasty healthy juice.

There is power in real juicing. You might say right now, that I am exaggerating, but I will tell you that it is true. It can heal, it can restore, and revitalize our physical body. It has so many real benefits that we cannot even imagine.

One benefit of juicing is, it gives us energy, when energy can nowhere be found. There are surely days where you really have to have energy because of so many appointments listed ahead. But sad to say, you don't know where those energies are. That is why juicing can help you. Juices from fruits like cucumber or celery, which is a recipe written below, is a good way to start up your day. These fruits and vegetables, are high in chlorophyll, that helps oxygenate the blood, increasing the brain function, and gives high energy. So, you can now, kick up your day, with your heads feeling good and energized!

That is just one benefit, there is still another. Great, right! If juicing gives you energy, it can also help you with sleeping. You have probably heard your mother or your doctor saying, "you need to have 8-10 hours of sleep". Even when you were still young, you've always known that. But some of you just can't, not because you won't, but you can't because of some sleep disorder, or some sleeping problem. It may also because you lack melatonin, a hormone that makes us sleep. Vitamin B6 is one of the main vitamins that produces melatonin. Many fruits, that can be juice, are vitamin B6 ready. Yes, there are a lot of supplements available in the counter, but there is no better than making it yourself.

Another benefit in juicing is, it can help us have a radiant and glowing skin like those celebrities we have seen on TV. Who doesn't want that? I believe that we all want that, a glossy radiant skin like those of celebrities. Do you know that famous celebrity, Salma Hayek, also believes in the power of juicing? She believes that juicing is cleansing. Well, it is true, because there are juices that remove toxins from our body, which is called detoxifying. These juices that are good for detox, are those who came from raw fruits and vegetables.

Raw fruits and vegetables are full of antioxidants. Antioxidants fight and neutralize the harmful effects of free radicals. These free radicals are like toxins, when not taken care of, it can cause illness, and damage to our skin cells. That is also why antioxidants are often used for skin care products. Since juicing came from raw fruits and vegetables, and are full of antioxidants, so this means, that juicing is a good way to look good and feel good. You want that, do you?

Not only because of the antioxidants that juicing has why you're having a great skin. But, also because, juicing is a good blood and liver cleanser. So, it doesn't only give you a healthy and natural glow of skin, but it can also heal chronic diseases that are caused by toxins in our body.

Juicing for weight loss. Probably many of you, are having a hard time in losing weight, especially when you love to eat. Juicing can help you with that. Aren't you happy? It can help you, by making your metabolism work faster, or by reducing your cravings. Many of us are not blessed with a boosting metabolism. But don't be discourage, we can aid you with that, there are fruits and vegetables that are good in making your metabolism work harder and faster. Like many others, juicing alone cannot make you lose weight, you still have to do your daily exercise, or do what your doctors tells you to do. These juicing recipes are just a helper that will help you be fit, and be healthy as possible.

Many people choose juicing as a way to a healthier life because of it's amazing benefits. The benefits of the fruits and vegetables itself, are also another benefit of juicing.

There are those who chose juicing because, they do not like to eat the whole fruit or the whole vegetable, because it doesn't taste pretty. Unlike in juicing, you can add other natural flavors from other fruits or vegetables that will complement each other, and will make its taste satisfactory. Besides, the nutrients aren't different. The vitamins that are in the whole fruit, can also be found in the juiced fruit.

Another great thing about juicing is that it is inexpensive compared to other manufactured juices, where you cannot even be sure if it is really natural or not. Also, it is so easy to make. You'll just have to chop some ingredients, or if you want, you can put them directly in your juicer or in any machine for juicing, and you're ready to go. You have now a cup of healthy fruity veggies in your hands.

Chapter 3

Are You Getting What You Need

Fruits and vegetables have different vitamins. But what exactly are these vitamins, and what does it do? Why do you have to know these things? Why, because you have to know what you are putting inside your body, and take track if you are getting what it needs. Because what you put inside is what you are on the outside.

Vitamin A, also known as Retinol, is recognized for its significance to have good eyesight. But not only that, but it is also used to maintain healthy skin. If you're having a problem of aging, vitamin A is good for you, because it reduces the growth of wrinkles in your face. It helps prevent dead skin cells and reduce the amount of oil in your skin. That's why sometimes, doctors recommend it to teenagers to treat acne. Vitamin A can be found in dark green leafy vegetables and yellow vegetables like pumpkin or squash. It can also be in deep or bright-colored fruits, like carrots and papayas.

The B-vitamin Family. B-vitamin is made up of eight different vitamins that work together to maintain the functioning of the body in a healthy manner. All of them are water-soluble. They are the ones responsible for the body's metabolic system, enhancing the function of the nervous system, and strengthening the immune system. They are all also good for energy boosting. They help the body to convert the fats, and the carbs that it has, into energy. That is why foods rich in B-vitamins are necessary for every breakfast, to help you all day. But the same with other vitamins, the B-vitamin family still functions individually in the body.

Vitamin B1 or Thiamin is best when it comes to our brain and nervous system's health. It is often called as an "anti-stress" vitamin, because of its ability to improve the capacity of the brain to withstand stressful situations. Beans and seeds are the most common source of thiamin, but it can also be found in vegetables like asparagus and potatoes, and fruits like watermelon and pineapple.

Vitamin B2, the second B-vitamin, also known as Riboflavin, is an excellent antioxidant. Antioxidants are the ones who helps in preventing diseases because this aid fights free radicals or toxins that are harmful to your body. Since it is an excellent antioxidant, it is also good and is best in helping you have a glowing and radiant skin. The best sources for Riboflavin are spinach, broccoli, and other green leafy vegetables

Vitamin B3, the third B-vitamin, also known as Niacin or Nicotinic Acid. This vitamin helps in lowering blood sugar, which is a great thing for people who have diabetes. It also helps improves memory, and reduce the risk of cardiovascular diseases, and balances cholesterol levels and triglycerides. So, vitamin B3 is best for older adults or those who are suffering from heart issues. Vitamin B3 is commonly found in starchy vegetables like potato and asparagus, and citrus fruits like grapefruit and oranges.

Vitamin B5, which is also called Pantothenic acid, the fifth B-vitamin discovered. It is a vitamin that helps relieves the cause of asthma, autism, and Parkinson's disease. Just like the Vitamin B1, it also helps lessen stress, and other mental problems like depression and anxiety, by regulating the hormones that cause these. This vitamin can be found in fruits like avocado, strawberries, and corn, and in vegetables like cauliflower and broccoli.

Vitamin B6 or other called as pyridoxine. These vitamins are most beneficial for ladies who are in their period. B6 is essential for balancing hormonal changes in the woman, and helps relieves premenstrual and menstrual discomfort and pain. Fruits like bananas and watermelons, and starchy vegetables like zucchini, potatoes, and pumpkin, are excellent sources of Vitamin B6.

Next is, Vitamin B9, also known as folic acid. This vitamin is essential for the formation of hemoglobin in our blood. It also helps produce and maintain new cells; that is why most doctors recommend pregnant women to take folic acid vitamins. Vitamin B9 are commonly found in spinach, asparagus, lentils, and in green leafy vegetables.

Vitamin C or Ascorbic Acid. Many of you have already heard about this vitamin. It is the most popular vitamin, especially for kids. Most mothers gave their children this vitamin to reduce the chances of their children to get colds or fever. What most people know about this vitamin is, it can help improve our immune system and help us not get sick. It is what people look first when they are feeling the first signs of cold. Few only knows that vitamin C is also great in developing bones, and maintaining healthy teethes and gums. Aside from these, vitamin C has still a lot to give; one is, it is important in wound healing. It also works to treat various infections, diabetes, heart diseases, and high blood pressures, and many others. So, as much as the kids needed vitamin C to help them strengthen their immune system, so as the adults. You probably know where this vitamin can be seen, yes! You're right! Vitamin C are commonly found in citrus fruits like oranges and lemons. But they can also be found in fruits like pineapple, strawberries, and kiwi, and in vegetables like broccoli, Brussel sprouts, and kale.

Vitamin D. There are who says that Vitamin D is not a vitamin. They say it is a steroid hormone that is made inside the body. But, they still consider it as a vitamin because it can still be obtained from other sources like fruits and vegetables. What does it do? Vitamin D like any other vitamins also has a lot of works to do, but it plays a great role especially in bone health. It also helps treats rickets, diabetes, tooth decay, and prevents osteoporosis. Vitamin D is often called as a sunshine vitamin because unlike any other vitamins; its sources are not commonly found in foods but the sun. The best way to develop this vitamin is by spending a few minutes out in our house.

Vitamin E or another term for it is Tocopherol. Research shows that people with high intakes of this vitamin are more protected from old-age related problems like Alzheimer's disease and menopause. It is also often used as anti-aging properties and protects against heart diseases, painful menstrual cycles, and brain malfunction, and it also improves blood circulation. Common sources of Vitamin E are from fruits like tomatoes and apples, and in any green vegetables like kale and asparagus.

Vitamin K, also called as Neonatal, is a vitamin that is important to avoid excessive bleeding. It plays an important role especially in blood clotting, but it is also necessary for building strong bones and in preventing heart diseases and cancer. Consuming vitamin K-rich foods can also help reduce infection, and restore oral health. People who have a history of cardiovascular disease and osteoporosis are highly recommended to add vitamin K in their diet. Vitamin K's best sources are in green leafy vegetables like Kale and in fruits like apples, avocados, and peaches.

If you are trying to lose weight, it is best for you to eat foods with high fiber. You might have probably heard about this thing, but what really is fiber? To easily explain it, fiber is what makes us feel full. For example, you will feel more satisfied if you have eaten a meal with 250 calories and 10 grams of fiber, than if you have eaten a meal with the same calories but no fiber. So, it will be longer for you to feel hungry again after eating a meal. That is how fiber helps you in losing weight.

Fiber also does other beneficial things, depending on whether it is soluble or insoluble. Soluble fiber slows down digestion by the absorption of fats and sugars. That is why soluble fiber is helpful in preventing and managing diabetes, and in lowering high cholesterols. Good sources of soluble fiber are fruits and vegetables like apples, oranges, and carrots.

While, insoluble fiber help food passes more quickly through the intestines. It also offers a lot of benefits to intestinal health, including constipation. So, if you are having a problem in controlling your bowel movements, adding more of it can help you get things moving. Fruits like avocados, bananas, and raspberries; and vegetables like broccoli and beets are good sources of insoluble fiber.

Keep in mind that too much of good things can be a bad thing, so a balanced diet is recommended for you to stay healthy as possible.

Chapter 4

Juice for a Glowing and Radiant Skin

Sweet Mango Juice

Yield: 2 Servings

Ingredients:

- 3 ripe mangoes
- 2 cucumbers
- 1 cup of pineapple chunks

Preparation:

- Peel the mangoes, and slice them into cubes.
- Peel the cucumbers, and slice them into thick slices.
- Add the mangoes, cucumbers, and pineapple into the juicer.
- Let the juicer blend for half a minute, and then press to extract the juice from the fruits.
- Transfer the juice into a glass.
- Serve and enjoy!

Benefits:

"Mangos are not just sweet fruits it also contains a lot of healthy things in it. Like Vitamin A and Beta-Carotene that will rejuvenate your skin. It contains a lot of antioxidants that will prevent toxins and harmful diseases from entering your body especially your skin. So if you want to keep you face and skin nice and clean then this is a great drink for you."

Nutritions:

Calories 148

Vitamins Present: Vitamin A, Vitamin B1, B5, B6, Vitamin C, Vitamin K.

Kale Green Juice

Yield: 1-2 Servings

Ingredients:

- 5 large kale leaves
- 2 cucumbers
- 1 lemon
- 2 lime
- 1 apple
- 1-inch ginger root
- 2 ribs celery

Preparation:

1. Wash properly all the fruits and vegetables.
2. Add them all into the juicer, and press until all juice is extracted.
3. Serve immediately.
4. (optional) Add ice.

Benefits:

"Kale leaves are one of the green leafy vegetables that are great especially when it comes to skin care. It is because Kale leaves are rich in Vitamin A and C which are great tools for skin maintenance. For the cucumber, it will help you stay hydrated. If you have acne or any skin conditions, your colon may be stocked up. Kale and Cucumber will surely help you by inducing a bowel movement, and flushes out the toxins out to your body."

Nutritions:

Calories 123

Vitamins Present: Vitamin A, Vitamin B1, B2, B3, B5, Vitamin C, Vitamin K.

Beet-Apple Juice

Yield: 1-2 Servings

Ingredients:

- 2 medium beets
- 1 apple
- 3 medium carrots

Preparation:

1. First, juice the beets, follow by the apples, and lastly the carrots.
2. Stir to combine well the fruit and vegetables.
3. Transfer to a glass, and serve immediately.

Benefits:

"Beets are fully packed with nutrients necessary for a healthy glowing skin. They are good liver and blood cleansers, and so as apples. Apples are known to be the healthiest fruit. You have probably heard the saying, "an apple a day keeps the doctors away," but have you know that apples are also excellent when it comes to skin? Apples' benefits for skin: It cleanses, as well as hydrates your skin; It provides additional protection from the rays of the sun; regular intake of apples helps eliminate your fine lines and wrinkles, and much more."

Nutritions:

Calories 120

Vitamins Present: Vitamin A, Vitamin B1, B2, B3, B5, B6, B9, Vitamin C, Vitamin E, and Vitamin K.

Pineapple Pear Juice

Yield: 1 Serving

Ingredients:

- 4 pineapple spears
- 1 pear

Preparation:

1. Slice pear into quarters.
2. Add pineapple and pear into the juicer, and press the fruits in the juicer until no more juice is extracted.
3. Serve immediately, and enjoy!

Benefits:

"Pineapple is like a storehouse for bromelain, vitamin C, and antioxidants, which are beneficial in the prevention of acne, sun damaged, and uneven skin tone. The vitamin C in the pineapple gives a healing touch to those who have sensitive and inflamed skin. While, Pear fruits are also excellent to treat oily skin, and makes skin moisturized for a long time. So, both pineapple and pear fruits are great fruits for healthy skin."

Nutritions:

Calories 152

Vitamins Present: Vitamin B1, B6, Vitamin C, and dietary fiber

Tomato Juice

Yield: 1 Serving

Ingredients:

- 4 medium tomatoes
- 1 cup sliced watermelon

Preparation:

1. Add the tomatoes and watermelon in the juicer.
2. Press until all juice is extracted.
3. Transfer juice mixture into a glass, and serve immediately.

Benefits:

"Tomatoes are the greatest sources of lycopene and is great for skin protection, especially when you will be going out in the sun for a long time, as it helps in protecting your skin from UV damage."

Nutritions:

Calories 118

Vitamins Present: Vitamin A, Vitamin B1, B6, Vitamin C, Vitamin E, and Vitamin K

Spinach Broccoli Juice

Yield: 2 Servings

Ingredients:

- ½ head of broccoli
- 3 cups full of spinach
- 2 apples
- 1 large cucumber
- ½ inch of ginger root

Preparation:

1. Wash all ingredients.
2. Cut the broccoli into chunks.
3. Slice the apples into quarters.
4. Slice thinly the cucumbers and ginger root, but not too thin.
5. Then, put all the ingredients in the juicer.
6. Let the juicer do its job, and press until all juice is extracted.
7. Serve immediately.

Benefits:

"Spinach and broccoli are great partners when it comes to healthy skin. Just like other vegetables, these green vegetables are wonderful sources for vitamins. They are rich in Vitamin A and Vitamin C that helps improve your complexion, and helps in skin repair, making your skin looking young, healthy and radiant."

Nutritions:

Calories 152

Vitamins Present: Vitamin A, Vitamin B1, B2, B6, Vitamin C, Vitamin E, and Vitamin K

Gooseberry Ginger Juice

Yield: 2 Servings

Ingredients:

- 2 Indian gooseberries
- 1 inch of ginger root
- 1 lemon
- A pinch of salt

Preparation:

1. Slice the gooseberries into chunks.
2. Slice thinly the ginger root or into quarters.
3. Add the sliced gooseberries and ginger root into the juicer.
4. Let it blend for half a minute, and press until all juice is extracted.
5. Add the lemon, taking out the seeds, then add the salt.
6. Stir until salt is dissolved or mixture is well combined.
7. Transfer it into a glass, and serve immediately.

Benefits:

"The gooseberries in this juice are full of Vitamin A, which helps in increasing the production of collagen, which is vital to keep your skin looking firm and radiantly beautiful. It is also a great antioxidant as well as the ginger root."

Nutritions:

Calories 138

Vitamins Present: Vitamin A, Vitamin B-Complex, Vitamin C, and Vitamin E

Chapter 5

Detox Juices

Tropical Pineapple Mint Juice

Yield: 2 Servings

Ingredients:

- 3 cups of mint leaves
- 1 cup of pineapple chunks
- 1 cucumber
- 2 stalks of celery
- 2 cups of spinach
- 1 lemon

Preparation:

1. Prepare your ingredients.
2. Chop or slice the ingredients into small pieces that will fit your juicer.
3. Juice first the mint leaves and the pineapple chunks together.
4. Next, juice together with the remaining ingredients.
5. Stir to combine well the juice extracts.
6. Serve immediately, and enjoy!

Benefits:

"Mint, pineapple, and cucumbers are all excellent ingredients for detox. They all are good helpers to remove toxins from your body and cleanse your liver. This juice is best taken when you have a long list of appointments. The mint in it will give you a refreshing feeling, the pineapple will help boost your energy, and the cucumber will help you stay hydrated."

Nutritions:

Calories 136

Vitamins Present: Vitamin A, Vitamin B1, B3, B6, Vitamin C, Vitamin K

Cellulite Eraser Grapefruit Juice

Yield: 1-2 Servings

Ingredients:

- 1 large grapefruit
- 2 large oranges
- 1 lime
- ½ inch of ginger root

Preparation:

1. Add the grapefruit, the oranges and the ginger root in your juicer.
2. Let the fruits be processed in the juicer, and press until all juice is extracted.
3. Transfer the juice mixture in a glass, and squeeze the lime.
4. Stir to mix.
5. Serve immediately, and enjoy!

Benefits:

"Grapefruits, Limes, Oranges and ginger roots are fruits that can help boost your immune system. All of them are great sources of vitamin C, which is important so that you will be able to avoid common and sometimes very serious diseases such as colds, flu, fever, etc. This is a great drink for those who get sick easily. If you're a parent, give this drink to your children to strengthen their immune system."

Nutritions:

Calories 136

Vitamins Present: Vitamin A, Vitamin B1, Vitamin B5, Vitamin C

Zucchini Green Juice

Yield: 2 Servings

Ingredients:

- 1 Zucchini
- 3 Pears
- 1/8 of fennel bulb
- 1 cup of broccoli florets
- A bunch of spinach

Preparation:

1. Wash thoroughly the ingredients.
2. Chop the zucchinis into thin slices.
3. Slice the pears into cubes.
4. Combine all ingredients in a juicer.
5. Process the ingredients until it can easily be pressed.
6. Press the mixture until all juice is extracted.
7. Transfer it into a glass, and serve immediately.

Benefits:

"A green juice, filled with vitamins and minerals to strengthen you for your day. This juice is a drink that can enable you to keep your nervous system healthy. Vitamin B2 is needed by the body because it cannot be produced by the human body, so it is a necessity, this drink is a great drink for all those green lovers out there. So, come on and try it out."

Nutritions:

Calories 152

Vitamins Present: Vitamin A, Vitamin B1, B2, B3, B6, Vitamin C, Vitamin K

Kiwi + Apple Juice

Yield: 2 Servings

Ingredients:

- 2 medium kiwi
- 1 medium apple
- 1 medium banana
- 1 lime
- ½ cup water

Preparation:

1. Slice the kiwi, apple, and banana into quarter slices.
2. Add the fruits into the juicer.
3. Let it blend for half a minute, and then press to extract the juices.
4. Transfer the juice mixture into a glass.
5. Squeeze the lime, and add the water.
6. Stir to combine well the mixture.
7. Add ice if desired. Serve and enjoy!

Benefits:

"Kiwi is like a superfood when it comes to detoxification. It helps prevent free radicals and helps to flush the toxins out to your body, which will also help improve your overall health. While apples, it is a nutritional powerhouse where vitamins are stored. When both are combined as juice, you will be amazed of its overall benefits."

Nutritions:

Calories 135

Vitamins Present: Vitamin A, Vitamin B6, Vitamin C, Vitamin E, Vitamin K

Pineapple Lime Juice

Yield: 2 Servings

Ingredients:

- 6 pineapple wedges
- 4 limes
- 2 lemons
- 1 cup of water

Preparation:

1. Prepare the ingredients.
2. Slice the pineapples into wedges.
3. Slice the limes into halves, so as the lemons.
4. Add the pineapple wedges into the juicer, and juice until no more juice are extracted.
5. Transfer the juice extracted into a glass with water.
6. Squeeze in the lime and the lemons.
7. Stir well to combine, and add ice if desired.
8. Serve immediately, and enjoy!

Benefits:

"Pineapples, Limes, and Lemons are all great sources of Vitamin C. Vitamin C is not produced inside the human body so it is very necessary for you to have it. This drink will be able to supply you with your daily dose of vitamin c and in turn, it will be able to help protect your body from impure elements and common diseases."

Nutritions:

Calories 99

Vitamins Present: Vitamin B1, B3, B6, Vitamin C

Watermelon Citrus Juice

Yield: 2 Servings

Ingredients:

- 2 cups of watermelon cubes
- 1 lemon
- 1 lime
- 1 orange
- 1 small cucumber

Preparation:

1. Prepare all the ingredients.
2. Slice the watermelon into cubes.
3. Slice into halves the citrus fruits: lemon, lime, and orange.
4. Slice thinly the cucumber.
5. Add the watermelon and the cucumber into the juicer.
6. Press to extract the juices from the fruits.
7. Squeeze in also the citrus fruits.
8. Press again the juicer until no more juice can be extracted.
9. Transfer into a glass. Serve immediately, and enjoy!

Benefits:

"This drink is good for those people who wants to keep in shape, and stay hydrated and energized in their workout. Watermelons are a great source of hydration because it is 92% water, and it contains a lot of Vitamins to help you detoxify your body. Also, lemons and limes are a great source of energy when you are feeling fatigued. So, take this drink if you're going out to the gym."

Nutritions:

Calories 103

Vitamins Present: Vitamin A, Vitamin B1, B6, Vitamin C, Vitamin E, and Vitamin K

Ginger Lemonade

Yield: 1-2 Servings

Ingredients:

- 4 lemons
- 2-inch of ginger root
- 4 Tbsp. of honey
- 1 cup water

Preparation:

1. Wash well the lemons and ginger root.
2. Mince the ginger root, and slice the lemons into halves.
3. Add the minced ginger root into the juicer.
4. Blend for 10 seconds, or until there will be a juice that can be extracted from the ginger root when pressed.
5. Add the lemon, and press again until all juice is extracted.
6. Pour juice into a glass with water.
7. Add the honey, and stir well to combine.
8. Serve immediately, and enjoy!

Benefits:

"Fill yourself up with energy with this drink. This drink will be able to help you finish your workout and exercises regiment without making you fatigued. It is a great supply of Vitamin C and energy giving minerals. Lemons are often sucked on by athletes in half times. So evidently you can stay on the move always and be kept awake all the time."

Nutritions:

Calories 53

Vitamins Present: Vitamin B1, B2, B3, B5, B6, Vitamin C, Vitamin E

Chapter 6

Juice to Lose Weight

Green Chia Juice

Yield: 1-2 Servings

Ingredients:

- 3 collard greens
- 1 large cucumber
- 2 Fuji apples
- 1 head of romaine lettuce
- 1 lime
- 1 Tbsp. Chia seeds

Preparation:

1. Wash properly all the fruits and vegetables.
2. Slice cucumber into thin slices.
3. Slice Fuji apples into chunks.
4. Peel off the leaves of the romaine lettuce.
5. Put all the ingredients into the juicer, except for the chia seeds.
6. Juice until all juice is extracted.
7. Transfer juice mixture in a glass, and then add chia seeds.
8. Serve immediately, and enjoy!

Benefits:

"This green juice has a nice combination of nutrients, and by drinking this juice, you are giving your body the right vitamins, and helping your metabolism to work faster. So, you will not just lose some weight, you will also gain vitamins that your body needs."

Nutritions:

Calories 125

Vitamins Present: Vitamin A, Vitamin B1, B2, B3, B5, B6, Vitamin C, Vitamin E, Vitamin K

Minty Citrus Juice

Yield: 2 Servings

Ingredients:

- 1 Pink Grapefruit
- 2 oranges
- 1 bunch of mint leaves
- 1 head of romaine lettuce

Preparation:

1. Wash all ingredients with clean water.
2. Peel the grapefruit and the oranges.
3. Add together all the ingredients into the juicer.
4. Let it juice, until all juice is extracted.
5. Transfer it into a glass, and add ice.
6. Serve immediately, and enjoy!

Benefits:

"This minty drink will help you lose weight. Why? You probably all know that sweets provide a lot of calories in our body, that we sometimes do not need, and there are really times that we are craving for something sweet and good. But, we don't have to worry about our cravings. Why spend money wandering over to those candy aisle, when you can make this minty citrus juice, not only it is filled with nutrients, but it is also low in calorie, and the mint added, also takes part by aiding your digestion."

Nutritions:

Calories 84

Vitamins Present: Vitamin A, Vitamin B1, B2, B3, B5, B6, Vitamin C

Red Cabbage Flax Juice

Yield: 1-2 Servings

Ingredients:

- 1 medium head of red cabbage
- 1 large cucumber
- 1 apple
- 1 lemon
- 1 Tbsp. flaxseed, ground

Preparation:

1. Wash all the ingredients thoroughly, especially the red cabbage.
2. Chop the red cabbage into quarters.
3. Chop the cucumber into thick slices.
4. Slice the apples into chunks.
5. After chopping or slicing the cabbage, cucumber and apple, add them together into the juicer.
6. Blend it for half a minute, and then press to extract the juices from the fruits and vegetables.
7. Transfer the extracted juice into a glass, and then squeeze the lemon, straining the seeds, and stir well to combine.
8. Add lastly the flax seeds. Stir again to mix.

9. Serve immediately, and enjoy!

Benefits:

"Red cabbage, the highlight of this recipe is a great way to prevent free radicals from entering your body. This drink will help you prevent cancer and heart diseases. This drink is also low calorie so those that wants to keep in shape while staying healthy this drink is a great choice. This is the drink that will help you stay fit and also stay healthy."

Nutritions:

Calories 212

Vitamins Present: Vitamin A, Vitamin B1, B2, B3, B5, B9, Vitamin C, Vitamin E, Vitamin K

Beet and Celery Juice

Yield: 1-2 Servings

Ingredients:

- 2 medium-size beet
- 10 celery stalks
- 2 bunch of cilantro
- 2 cup of chopped spinach
- 1 tsp. of sea salt

Preparation:

1. Wash thoroughly with water the beet, celery stalks, cilantro, and spinach.
2. Prepare the Ingredients: Cube the beets; cut celery stalks into chunks; and chop cilantro into medium sizes.
3. Add them all together in the juicer, and then blend for half a minute, and then extract the juice from the blended ingredients.
4. Transfer the extracted juice into a glass, and then add sea salt.
5. Stir until salt is dissolved.
6. Serve immediately, and enjoy!

Benefits:

"Great drink for those who wants to build their bodies and also those who wants to keep their bowels feel good. It is rich in potassium that helps build your muscles, and fibers that help your bowel movement to stay good. Also, if you like the flavor of beets then this is a great drink for you!"

Nutritions:

Calories 56

Vitamins Present: Vitamin A, Vitamin B1, B2, B3, B5, B6, Vitamin C, Vitamin E, Vitamin K

Pomegranate and Lychee Juice

Yield: 2 Servings

Ingredients:

- 2 cups of deseeded lychee
- 2 cups of pomegranates
- 1 lemon

Preparation:

1. Peel and then deseed the lychees.
2. Add all the ingredients in the juicer.
3. Press the juicer to extract the juice from the fruits.
4. Transfer the juice mixture into a glass.
5. Serve immediately, and enjoy!

Benefits:

"A great drink for those who wants to keep the production of the blood in their bodies stay good. It contains antioxidants that prevent harmful toxins from entering your body backed with Vitamin C that strengthens your immune system and also a big necessity for your body. Such an easy drink to make and very healthy for a very low ingredient count drink."

Nutritions:

Calories 138

Vitamins Present: Vitamin B2, B3, B6, Vitamin C, Vitamin K

Spinach and Apple Juice

Yield: 1-2 Servings

Ingredients:

- 3 medium-size apples
- 2 cups of chopped spinach
- ½ of red lettuce
- 1 lemon
- ¼ tsp. cayenne pepper
- 1 tsp. salt

Preparation:

1. Wash thoroughly the apples, spinach, lettuce, and lemon.
2. Chop the apples into cubes.
3. Peel the leaves of the red lettuce.
4. Add the first four ingredients into the juicer.
5. Let it blend for 30 seconds, and then press the juicer to extract the juices from the fruits.
6. Transfer the extracted juice into a glass.
7. Add the cayenne pepper and salt.
8. Serve immediately, and enjoy!

Benefits:

"An apple a day keeps the doctors away is not just a saying but a fact. It can reduce the risk of diabetes, stroke, breast cancer and bad cholesterol levels. It can also prevent dementia keeping your brain healthy. Cayenne pepper is a great spice with a lot of benefits one is a detoxifying agent keeping toxins away. A great and easy drink for those who wants to stay healthy."

Nutritions:

Calories 124

Vitamins Present: Vitamin A, Vitamin B1, B2, B3, B5, B6, B9, Vitamin C, Vitamin E, and Vitamin K

Kale Apple Juice

Yield: 2-3 Servings

Ingredients:

- 10 Kale Leaves
- 4 Green Apples
- 4 Carrots
- 4 Celery stalks

Preparation:

1. Wash the fruits and vegetables thoroughly.
2. Chop the apples, carrots, and celery stalks into medium bits, just enough sizes to fit your juicer.
3. Add them, the kale leaves, apples, carrots, and celery stalks to your juicer.
4. Juice them all together, when there is no more juice is extracted, transfer the juice into a glass.
5. Serve immediately, and enjoy!

Benefits:

"Kale is one of those green leafy veggies who has surprisingly a lot of benefits, and one is that it can aid in weight loss! Did you know that kale has zero fat and has a low amount of calorie? It also has high fiber content, which helps in aiding digestion and eliminating wastes. So, if you love greens and you'd love to lose some weight, then make this juice, and drink it early in the morning on an empty stomach."

Nutritions:

Calories 157

Vitamins Present: Vitamin A, Vitamin B1, B2, B5, B6, Vitamin C, Vitamin E, and Vitamin K

Chapter 7

Cleanse Your Body with Juicing

Spiced Berry Juice

Yield: 2 Servings

Ingredients:

- 2 cups of strawberries
- 2 cup of raspberries
- 1 cup of dandelion leaves
- 1 small chili

Preparation:

1. Remove the skin and the seeds of the chili.
2. Add the strawberries and the raspberries in the juicer.
3. Let it juice for a minute, until all juice from the fruits is extracted.
4. Transfer to a glass, and then stir well.
5. Serve immediately, and enjoy!

Benefits:

"Strawberries are one the fruits that are excellent sources of antioxidant. We all know that antioxidants are great for cleansing, for they neutralize the effects of harmful radicals in our body, and help the liver to carry out its cleansing functions. The chili in the juice also helps in giving a refreshing flavor in your drink. So, this is a great drink if you are feeling constipated."

Nutritions:

Calories 125

Vitamins Present: Vitamin B5, B6, Vitamin C, and Vitamin K

Papaya Tropical Juice

Yield: 2-3 Servings

Ingredients:

- 1 medium-size ripe papaya
- 2 cups of fresh pineapple chunks
- 2 medium kiwi
- An inch of ginger root
- ½ cup of fresh coconut water

Preparation:

1. Peel and then chop the papaya into medium chunks.
2. Slice thinly the ginger root.
3. Slice into quarters the kiwi.
4. Add together the papaya, pineapple, and ginger root into the juicer.
5. Let it blend, and then press the juicer to extract the juice from the fruits.
6. Transfer into a glass, and then add the coconut water.
7. Stir well to combine, and add ice if desired.
8. Serve immediately, and enjoy!

Benefits:

"This drink is packed with antioxidants and amino acids that help your body keep toxins out and build up your body's muscles. A great drink for people who love working out and those who want to keep their bodies in shape. This drink also enables you to avoid chances of stroke. Potassium also helps your body build the necessary muscles that you need to avoid unnecessary injuries. So, bodybuilders and people who want to stay fit come and give it a try."

Nutritions:

Calories 169

Vitamins Present: Vitamin A, Vitamin B1, B5, B6, Vitamin C, Vitamin E, and Vitamin K

Carrot + Sweet Potato + Beet Juice

Yield: 1-2 Servings

Ingredients:

- 2 Beet Roots
- 10 Carrots
- 1 medium-size Sweet Potato

Preparation:

1. Chop the beet roots, the carrots and, the sweet potato into chunks.
2. Combine them together in the juicer.
3. Blend for a minute, until it can be press.
4. Press the juicer to extract the juices from the ingredients.
5. Transfer to a glass. Serve immediately, and enjoy!

Benefits:

"Carrots are great ingredients that contain a lot of antioxidants that can cleanse your body of harmful toxins. It also contains Vitamin A that keeps your eyes clear and your bones grow. It also supports the Immune system to keep diseases away from your body. So stay healthy now with this easy to make drink."

Nutritions:

Calories 169

Vitamins Present: Vitamin A, Vitamin B1, B2, B3, B5, B6, Vitamin C, Vitamin E, Vitamin K

Carrot Cleanser Juice

Yield: 2-3 Servings

Ingredients:

- 4 Carrots
- 2 Red Apples
- 1 Kiwi
- 2 Stalks of celery
- ½ Cucumber
- 1 Inch fresh Ginger Root
- 1 Lemon

Preparation:

1. Wash thoroughly the ingredients.
2. Chop the carrots and apples into cubes.
3. Slice the kiwi into half.
4. Chop the celery stalks and the cucumber into medium bits.
5. Mince the ginger root.
6. Add all the ingredients into the juicer.
7. Let it blend for a while, or until it can already be pressed.
8. Press the juicer, and let the juice be extracted.
9. Transfer the juice into a glass.
10. Serve immediately, and enjoy!

Benefits:

"Carrots are full of beta carotene and antioxidants to keep your body clean and healthy. Not to mention apples are one of the best fruits that help clean your body. It has a lot of fibers and also a lot of antioxidants so that not only your body and blood is clean but also your colon will be as healthy."

Nutritions:

Calories 106

Vitamins Present: Vitamin A, Vitamin B1, B2, B3, B5, B6, B9, Vitamin C, Vitamin E, and Vitamin K

Clementine Juice

Yield: 2 Servings

Ingredients:

- 4 Clementine
- 2 Apples
- 1 stick of cinnamon
- 1 lemon

Preparation:

1. Slice clementine and lemon into half, and squeeze to juice, and strain the seeds.
2. Chop apples into chunks, and juice them in the juicer.
3. Combine all the juices of the fruits into a glass.
4. Stir using the cinnamon stick.
5. Let the cinnamon stick soak in the juice for 10 minutes, before serving.
6. Serve and enjoy!

Benefits:

"Citruses are great fruits to cleanse your body. As Clementine is a citrus it is a good way to clean the body. Clementine also has Vitamin C which is a vitamin that the body needs to prevent scurvy. Vitamin C cannot be produced inside of the human body so that is why it is a necessity. Combine it with lemons and apples then you have a very citrusy and sweet drink."

Nutritions:

Calories 148

Vitamins Present: Vitamin A, Vitamin B1, B2, B3, B5, B9, Vitamin C, Vitamin E, Vitamin K

Apple Strawberry Juice

Yield: 2 Servings

Ingredients:

- 4 cups Strawberries
- 2 Red Apples
- 2 Cucumbers

Preparation:

1. Remove the tops of the strawberries.
2. Chop the apples into chunks.
3. Slice the cucumbers into thick slices.
4. Add all the ingredients in the juicer.
5. Let it blend for half a second, and press to juice the fruits.
6. Transfer the juice in a glass.
7. Serve immediately, and enjoy!

Benefits:

"Strawberries and apples are full of antioxidants that cleanse the body. They are also sweet fruits that are good to eat. Apples have many documented benefits which include preventing cancer, lowering calorie levels and also preventing hypertension.

Strawberries also have dietary fibers that can help you cleanse your colon. So make and enjoy your drink."

Nutritions:

Calories 196

Vitamins Present:

Vitamin A, Vitamin B1, B2, B3, B5, B6, B9, Vitamin C, Vitamin E, Vitamin K

Chapter 8

Juice and Have a Good Eyesight

Carrot + Orange Juice

Yield: 4 servings

Ingredients:

- 2 organic carrots
- 8 organic oranges

Preparation:

1. Peel carrots, and slice into cubes.

2. Slice oranges into halves.

3. Add the cubed carrots into the juicer, and squeeze the oranges.

4. Press the juicer until all juice of the carrots and oranges are extracted.

5. Transfer into a large glass.

Benefits:

"We all know that carrots contain Vitamin A that can help your eyesight stay clear. But did you know that it contains antioxidants to help you clean your body and keep toxins away. This drink also contains oranges that help with keeping common diseases away.

So if you want healthy eyes and a clean body you can make this drink now."

Nutritions:

Calories 103

Vitamins Present: Vitamin A, Vitamin B1, Vitamin B2, Vitamin B3, Vitamin B5, Vitamin B6, Vitamin C, Vitamin K

Watercress + Carrot Juice

Yield: 2 Servings

Ingredients:

- 1 cup of watercress chopped
- 3 medium-size carrots
- ½ cup of cilantro
- ½ cup of spinach
- 2 Roma tomatoes
- A pinch of salt

Preparation:

1. Wash thoroughly the vegetables.
2. Chop carrots into dice-size.
3. Chop all other vegetables, and throw them directly to the juicer.
4. Turn on juicer, and process everything together, and press until all juice is extracted.
5. Transfer juice in a glass.
6. Add ice if desired. Serve immediately, and enjoy!

Benefits:

"Watercress is a good ingredient to help restore your energy and adding the carrots helps keep your eyes on the clear side. This is also a great drink for people who like working out while also keeping your eyes well. This drink is also a refreshing because it has a lot of greens in. So what are you waiting for green lovers!"

Nutritions:

Calories 73

Vitamins Present: Vitamin A, Vitamin B1, B2, B5, B6, Vitamin C, Vitamin E, Vitamin K

Carrot Ginger Apple Juice

Yield: 2 Servings

Ingredients:

- 4 Carrots
- 2-inch of ginger
- 3 Green Apples
- 2 stalks of celery
- 1 cup of chopped endive
- 1 cup of chopped parsley

Preparation:

1. Chop carrots, apples, and celery into medium bits.
2. Crush ginger and slice into half.
3. Add the ingredients into the juicer.
4. Blend it for a minute, and then press the juicer to extract the juice.
5. Transfer the extracted juice into a glass.
6. Serve immediately, and enjoy!

Benefits:

"Vitamin A and beta-carotene are great nutrients that can help your eyes and all of these are contained in carrots. Also, the ginger is a great ingredient that has antioxidants that can clean your body of wastes and toxins. Ginger can also treat nausea so for those who are groggy in the morning this is a great drink."

Nutritions:

Calories 150

Vitamins Present: Vitamin A, Vitamin B1, B2, B3, B5, B6, Vitamin C, Vitamin E, Vitamin K

Peachy Carrot Juice

Yield: 2-3 Servings

Ingredients:

- 5 medium-size Peaches
- 14 Carrots
- 3 Fresh basil leaves
- 1 lemon

Preparation:

1. Wash thoroughly the ingredients with clean water to remove harmful chemicals, if there are any.
2. Chop peaches and carrots into medium-size cubes.
3. Chop or mince the basil leaves.
4. Slice the lemon into half.
5. Add the peaches, carrots, and basil leaves into your juicer.
6. Blend for half a minute, and press the juicer to extract the juice from the fruits.
7. Transfer the juice into a glass, and squeeze lemon, straining the seeds.
8. Serve immediately, and enjoy!

Benefits:

"Peaches contains potassium which is great for building muscles. Also, it also contains carrots that contain Vitamin A which helps your eyes. One of the great things about this drink is you can shape your body while maintaining your eyes. This is a great drink for all the body builders out there so why not give it a try."

Nutritions:

Calories 196

Vitamins Present: Vitamin A, Vitamin B1, B2, B3, B5, B6, Vitamin C, Vitamin E, Vitamin K

Carrot Zest with Red Pepper

Yield: 2 Servings

Ingredients:

- 10 Carrots
- 4 oranges
- 1 lemon
- 2 red bell peppers
- 1-inch of ginger

Preparation:

1. Wash thoroughly the ingredients with clean water to remove harmful chemicals, if there are any.
2. Chop the carrots into medium-sized chunks or cubes.
3. Peel the oranges and lemon.
4. Deseed the red bell peppers, and slice them into halves.
5. Crush the ginger.
6. Add all the ingredients in the juicer, and blend them together.
7. Press the juicer to extract the juice from the ingredients.
8. Transfer the extracted juice into a glass.
9. Serve immediately, and enjoy!

Benefits:

"Carrots, such amazing ingredients for the eyes but not only for the eyes but it is also a great root vegetable for digestion because it contains fibers that can help clean the colon. Plus the zesty taste from the lemons and the oranges can help freshen up your day. With a hint of ginger and peppers to add a more flavorful kick, this is a great drink for a morning rise."

Nutritions:

Calories 210

Vitamins Present: Vitamin A, Vitamin B1, B2, B3, B5, B6, Vitamin C, Vitamin E, Vitamin K

Carrot Beet Juice

Yield: 2 Servings

Ingredients:

- 8 carrots
- 1 beet root
- 1 apple
- 1-inch ginger
- 1 orange
- 1 sweet potato

Preparation:

1. Wash all ingredients with clean water to remove if there are any toxins.
2. Chop carrots, apples, and sweet potatoes into quarters.
3. Slice beet root into half.
4. Peel the orange.
5. Crush the ginger and slice into half.
6. Add all the ingredients in the juicer, and process it for a minute.
7. Press the juicer to extract the juices.
8. Transfer the juice into a glass.
9. Serve immediately, and enjoy!

Benefits:

"Boost your Vitamin C and protect your body from common illness with beets. This juice contains beets and oranges that give you your daily dose of Vitamin C. The citrusy taste of the oranges really makes the taste of this drink so much better. It also contains carrots that have Vitamin A to help your eyes stay clear."

Nutritions:

Calories 185

Vitamins Present:

Vitamin A, Vitamin B1, B2, B3, B5, B6, B9, Vitamin C, Vitamin E, Vitamin K

Chapter 9

Energy Boost

Minty Fruit Cocktail Juice

Yields: 2 Servings

Ingredients:

- 2 apples
- 2 oranges
- 1 cup of pineapple chunks
- 2 cups of watermelon
- 2 tsp. of lemon juice
- Fresh mint

Preparation:

1. Peel and then slice the apple.
2. Peel the orange and divide it.
3. Slice the watermelon into medium cubes and then seed it.
4. Juice both the apple and orange, then juice the pineapple.
5. Transfer the juice to the blender then add the watermelon, lemon juice, and mint.
6. Blend until smooth.
7. Transfer into a glass and add ice if desired.
8. Serve immediately, and enjoy!

Benefits:

"An apple a day keeps the doctor away is not just a phrase but a fact. Apples contains a lot of nutrients that can supply your body. The sugars in the apples also provides a natural energy boost. Combined with the taste of the oranges and lemons this drink is a great drink to start your day."

Nutritions:

Calories 212

Vitamins Present: Vitamin A, Vitamin B1, B2, B3, B5, B6, Vitamin C, Vitamin E, Vitamin K

Kale Green Juice with Tomatoes

Yield: 2 servings

Ingredients:

- 2 branches of kale
- 2 apples
- 1 cucumber
- 2 tomatoes

Preparation:

1. Wash all ingredients thoroughly.
2. Slice the tomato, apple, and cucumber into medium chunks.
3. Add all ingredients into the juicer.
4. Transfer it to glass and then stir.
5. Serve immediately, and enjoy!

Benefits:

"Kale is such an amazing ingredient that contains almost anything that your body needs from vitamin a to vitamin c. Mixing it with tomatoes that contain a lot of antioxidants make this a perfect drink for taking care of your body. Also with apples to supply you with the necessary energy and to balance out the taste."

Nutritions:

Calories 157

Vitamins Present: Vitamin A, Vitamin B1, B2, B3, B5, B6, Vitamin C, Vitamin E, Vitamin K

Pear + Red Cabbage

Yield: 2 servings

Ingredients:

- 2 medium-sized pears
- 1 red cabbage
- ½ cup lemon juice

Preparation:

1. Wash the pear thoroughly.
2. Slice the pears into chunks.
3. Peel 4 leaves off the red cabbage.
4. Add all the ingredients to the juicer.
5. Transfer the juice into a glass and stir.
6. Serve immediately, and enjoy!

Benefits:

"Pears contains a lot of sugars such as glucose and fructose that can give your body natural energy. It also has vitamin c and a lot of antioxidants to keep your body safe from toxins. Cleanse and energize your body with this drink now."

Nutritions:

Calories 145

Vitamins Present: Vitamin A, Vitamin B6, Vitamin C, Vitamin K

Celery and Beet Juice

Yield: 2 servings

Ingredients:

- 6 stalks of celery
- 1 green apple
- ½ of cucumber
- 1 beet

Preparation:

1. Wash all ingredients thoroughly.
2. Slice the green apple and the cucumber.
3. Add all the ingredients to the juicer. Add more cucumber if desired.
4. Transfer into the and stir gently.
5. Serve immediately, and enjoy!

Benefits:

"Celery contains a lot of Vitamins and minerals some of which gives you the energy to start your day. Celery also contains Vitamin C to protect the body from common illness. Added with cucumbers and beets surely makes this a healthy drink and an apple to balance its taste and flavor."

Nutritions:

Calories 74

Vitamins Present: Vitamin A, Vitamin B1, B2, B5, B6, Vitamin C, Vitamin K

Minty Papaya and Strawberry Juice

Yield: 2 servings

Ingredients:

- 1 cup of strawberries
- ½ of a large papaya
- Fresh mint

Preparation:

1. Wash all ingredients.
2. Cut the papaya into medium chunks.
3. Slice the stems off the strawberries
4. Add the strawberry and papaya into the juicer.
5. Transfer the juice into the and stir.
6. Place the mint on the top and add ice if desired.
7. Serve immediately, and enjoy!

Benefits:

"Strawberries and papaya are great ingredients if you love your drink mildly sweet. This drink is a great drink to enjoy with the family. This also has mint which can calm your digestion and extinguish your fatigue supplying you with energy. A great drink for those who love to enjoy it."

102

Nutritions:

Calories 107

Vitamins Present: Vitamin A, Vitamin B1, B2, B3, B6, Vitamin C

Vegetable Juice with Blueberry

Yields: 2 servings

Ingredients:

- 1 apple
- 1 cup of blueberry
- 1 stalk of broccoli
- 6 large carrots
- 1 tomato

Preparation:

1. Wash all ingredients thoroughly.
2. Peel and slice the apple.
3. Slice the carrots into medium cubes.
4. Slice the tomato.
5. Add all the ingredients to the juicer.
6. Transfer the juice into the and mix well.
7. Serve immediately, and enjoy!

Benefits:

"Apple, blueberry, broccoli, carrots and tomato, these ingredients contain a lot of vitamins and minerals that can help you start your day. These ingredients contain antioxidants that keep sickness away so that you will be full of energy every day. So try this drink now."

Nutritions:

Calories 205

Vitamins Present: Vitamin A, Vitamin B1, B2, B3, B5, B6, Vitamin C, Vitamin E, Vitamin K

Chapter 10

Lower Cholesterol

Peach Lemon Juice

Yield: 4 servings

Ingredients:

- 5 peaches
- 3 basil leaves
- 14 carrots
- ½ of lemon

Preparation:

1. Wash all ingredients.
2. Slice the carrots into cubes.
3. Slice the peaches into quarters.
4. Juice the basil leaves, lemon, peaches, and carrots in the respective order.
5. Transfer juice into the glass and mix well.
6. Serve immediately, and enjoy.

Benefits:

"Peaches contains no saturated fat or cholesterol. It is also low calorie so you do not need to worry about getting out of shape. If staying in shape while also having a great drink is what you want then this drink is for you. The peaches and carrots make a great taste. So try it right now!"

Nutritions:

Calories 146

Vitamins Present: Vitamin A, Vitamin B1, B2, B3, B5, B6, Vitamin C, Vitamin E, Vitamin K

Broccoli and Celery Juice

Yield: 2 servings

Ingredients:

- 3 stalks of celery
- 2 ½ cups of broccoli
- 1 cucumber
- 1 small ginger

Preparations:

1. Chop the celery and measure 2 ½ cup of chopped celery.
2. Chop the broccoli.
3. Slice the cucumber into chunks and measure 1 ½ of sliced cucumber.
4. Add all the ingredients to the juicer.
5. Extract the juice from all ingredients.
6. Transfer into the glass.
7. Serve immediately, and enjoy.

Benefits:

"Like Peaches, Broccoli contains no saturated fat or cholesterol. It is a great drink to keep healthy and to stay in shape. This drink not only is good for your body but it also tastes refreshing with all the greens in it. So stay fit and healthy with this drink."

Nutritions:

Calories 64

Vitamins Present: Vitamin A, Vitamin B1, B2, B3, B5, B6, Vitamin C, Vitamin E, Vitamin K

Cholesterol-Lowering Cocktail

Yield: 1-2 servings

Ingredients:

- 4 carrots
- 3 stalks of celery
- 1 broccoli
- 1 cucumber
- 1 green apple
- 1 kale leaf
- 1 lime

Preparation:

1. Scrub the sides of the carrot, remove its top, trim its end and then slice.
2. Peel the lime.
3. Slice all ingredients to fit into the juicer.
4. Add all ingredients and then juice until all juices are extracted.
5. Transfer into the and stir well.
6. Serve immediately, and enjoy!

Benefits:

"One of the ingredients celery contains dietary fibers that help with digestion and helps with your diet. It helps you keep your body healthy and fit. The kale leaves also help with digestion as well as many health benefits to list out. This is a great drink for those who wants to stay fit but enjoy a good drink as well."

Nutritions:

Calories 149

Vitamin Present: Vitamin A, Vitamin B1, B2, B5, B6, Vitamin C, Vitamin E, Vitamin K

Artichoke Juice

Yield: 1 Serving

Ingredients:

- 1 artichoke heart
- 2 stalks of celery
- ½ of a garlic head
- ½ glass of water

Preparation:

1. Steam the artichoke heart.
2. Mince the garlic head.
3. Stop steaming at desired perfection.
4. Place all ingredients including water to blender.
5. Blend well until smooth.
6. Transfer juice into the and add ice if desired.
7. Serve immediately, and enjoy!

Benefits:

"Controlling your cholesterol level is so easy with this drink thanks to artichokes. This vegetable helps with not only cholesterol but digestion as well. This drink also contains celery which has dietary fibers that help with colon cleansing.

Artichokes also has a lot of benefits on your liver. So stay healthy with this drink."

Nutritions:

Calories 58

Vitamins Present: Vitamin A, Vitamin B1, B2, B5, B6 B12, Vitamin C, Vitamin K

Low-Cholesterol Fruit Juice

Yield: 3-4 servings

Ingredients:

- 3 basil leaves
- 1 ½ cup of blueberries
- 2 pinches of cayenne pepper
- ½ of lime
- 5 cups of watermelon

Preparation:

1. Wash all ingredients thoroughly.
2. Place all ingredients into the juicer.
3. Juice until all juices are extracted.
4. Shake and stir it until well combined.
5. Transfer into the and add ice if desired.
6. Serve immediately, and enjoy!

Benefits:

"Stay low-calorie with this drink and keep in shape. Shaping the body is so much easier with this because this is a good and refreshing drink with just the right amount of calories. This drink also has lime and cayenne pepper to help regulate the toxins that come in your body. So try it out now."

Nutritions:

Calories 106

Vitamins Present: Vitamin A, Vitamin B1, B6, Vitamin C, Vitamin E, Vitamin K

Pineapple Lemon Juice

Yield: 4-5 servings

Ingredients:

- 4 cups of sliced pineapple
- 3 lemons
- ½ Tbsp. cinnamon
- 8 ½ cups of water
- 1 pinch of cloves

Preparation:

1. Place a pineapple and a glass of water in the blender. Blend it.
2. Extract juice from 3 lemons using a juicer.
3. Stir the lemon juice and spices into the remaining water and stir well.
4. Add the blended pineapple and the lemon juice mixture and stir until it becomes uniform.
5. Cool the juice in the refrigerator for a couple of hours.
6. Remove juice from the refrigerator at desired time.
7. Serve and enjoy!

Benefits:

"Pineapples contain the right nutrients and minerals to maintain your cholesterol levels. It is a great fruit for those who wants to keep their cholesterol in check. It would be much better as a drink mixed with lemons and many other ingredients to make it taste better. This is a great tasting drink that keeps you healthy so why not try it now!"

Nutritions:

Calories 107

Vitamin Present: Vitamin A, Vitamin B1, B2, B6, B12, Vitamin C, Vitamin D, Vitamin E, Vitamin K

Chapter 11
Juice for Digestion

Pear Juice

Yield: 2 Servings

Ingredients:

- 3 pears
- 4 stalks of celery
- 2-inch ginger
- 1 lemon

Preparation:

1. Wash all the ingredients properly.
2. Chop the pears into cubes.
3. Chop the celery into medium sizes.
4. Crush and divide the ginger into half.
5. Slice the lemon into half.
6. Add all the ingredients into the juicer.
7. Blend the ingredients for half a minute, and then press to extract the juice.
8. Transfer the juice into a glass.
9. Serve immediately, and enjoy!

Benefits:

"Pears are high fiber food that also gives you the necessary amount of nutrients to keep your body running. Fibers help to digest food and also keeps the colon clean. This drink can help you when you are constipated so try it out."

Nutritions:

Calories 183

Vitamins Present: Vitamin A, Vitamin B1, B2, B3, B5, B6, Vitamin C, Vitamin K

Pineapple Grapefruit Juice

Yield: 2 Servings

Ingredients:

- ½ of pineapple
- 2 yellow grapefruits
- 2 ruby grapefruits
- 2 carrots
- 2 lemon

Preparation:

1. Wash the ingredients properly.
2. Slice the pineapples into chunks.
3. Peel and slice the yellow and ruby grapefruits into quarters.
4. Peel and chop the carrots into cubes.
5. Slice the lemons into halves.
6. Add all the ingredients into the juicer.
7. Blend for half a minute, and then press to extract the juice.
8. Transfer juice into a glass, and give it a stir.
9. Serve immediately, and enjoy!

Benefits:

"Bromelain is a digestive enzyme that pineapple has. It is a mix of proteolytic enzymes. These enzymes help your stomach digest your food. It also helps your body absorb the nutrients in this food. Not only does this drink help your body digest the food it also helps it to absorb the food. So check it out now."

Nutritions:

Calories 204

Vitamins Present: Vitamin A, Vitamin B1, B2, B5, B6, Vitamin C, Vitamin K

Orange Aloe

Yield: 2 Servings

Ingredients:

- 4 oranges
- ½ cup juice of pure Aloe Vera
- A handful of spinach leaves

Preparation:

1. Wash the oranges and spinach leaves properly.
2. Peel the oranges and slice into halves.
3. Add all the ingredients into the juicer.
4. Blend for a minute, and then press to extract the juice.
5. Transfer the juice into a glass.
6. Serve immediately, and enjoy!

Benefits:

"Feeling bloated? Then this drink is right for you. Orange is a great fruit that helps the food in your stomach prevent from fermenting that causes gas. This drink also contains aloe that has enzymes that help with the overall digestion of food in the body. A great drink to try if you feel bloated and constipated a lot."

Nutritions:

Calories 123

Vitamins Present: Vitamin A, Vitamin B1, B2, B5, B6, Vitamin C, Vitamin E, Vitamin K

Cucumber Swiss Chard Juice

Yield: 2-3 Servings

Ingredients:

- 4 Cucumbers
- 16 leaves of Swiss Chard
- 2 cups of Pineapple chunks
- 1 lemon

Preparation:

1. Wash the ingredients properly.
2. Slice cucumbers into thick slices.
3. Add all the ingredients in the juicer.
4. Blend for a minute until it is ready to be press.
5. Press the juicer to extract the juice from the fruits and vegetables.
6. Transfer the extracted juice in a glass.
7. Serve immediately, and enjoy!

Benefits:

"Feeling constipated? Cucumber Swiss Chard Juice is the perfect combination for your digestive issues. It has an amazing source of Vitamin A and beta-carotene, which are excellent anti-inflammatory agents and antioxidants. It helps soothes your digestive tract that will help you in removing unwanted wastes in your body. So, feel refreshed with this swiss drink."

Nutritions:

Calories 165

Vitamins Present: Vitamin A, Vitamin B1, B2, B5, B6, Vitamin C, Vitamin E, Vitamin K

Orange Zucchini Juice

Yield: 2 Servings

Ingredients:

- 4 Zucchinis
- 4 oranges
- 1 head of lettuce
- 1 cup of pineapple chunks

Preparation:

1. Wash the ingredients properly to remove chemicals.
2. Chop the zucchinis and lettuce roughly into medium pieces.
3. Peel the oranges and slice into halves.
4. Add all the ingredients in the juicer.
5. Blend for a minute, and then press to extract the juice.
6. Transfer the juice into a glass.
7. Serve immediately, and enjoy!

Benefits:

"Zucchinis are recommended for digestive problems because it is hydrating and provides electrolytes and essential nutrients to the body. It is also very helpful as an anti-inflammatory remedy because it can help with ulcer. It is also easily digested because it is mostly water so for those who wants to digest food better then try this drink."

Nutritions:

Calories 175

Vitamins Present: Vitamin A, Vitamin B1, B5, B6, Vitamin C

Spicy Lime Juice

Yield: 2-3 Servings

Ingredients:

- 4 limes
- 1 jalapeno
- ½ of pineapple
- 2 Cucumbers
- 1 cup of chopped cilantro

Preparation:

1. Wash all the ingredients properly.
2. Peel the limes and slice them into halves.
3. Chop the pineapples into medium-sizes chunks.
4. Slice the cucumbers into thick slices.
5. Add all the ingredients in the juicer.
6. Blend for a minute, and then press to extract the juice.
7. Transfer the juice into a glass.
8. Serve immediately, and enjoy!

Benefits:

"Limes has a scent that stirs up the digestive properties in your mouth. It can help with the primary digestion before food comes to the stomach so it has great effects on your digestive system. This drink also contains Jalapenos that also helps with digestion. A spicy and refreshing drink that also helps with digestion why not try it now!"

Nutritions:

Calories 174

Vitamins Present: Vitamin A, Vitamin B1, B2, B3, B5, B6, Vitamin C, Vitamin E, Vitamin K

CONCLUSION

Thank you again for downloading this book.

I hope this book has provided you with the details and guidance in preparing your juices for your objectives and maybe discover a favorite or two juices that you like it very much. Do share it with us by posting a short review on Amazon. We love to hear from you.

Juicing is a great way to start your weight loss and a healthy journey. The delicious recipes that we share cover other areas of interests such as juicing for a glowing skin, getting an energy boost when you are tired and not just about weight loss. However, they are by no means comprehensive. Be adventurous and try different variations.

What next?

You have to commit yourself to adopt a healthy lifestyle that will keep you fit, lean and be mindfulness about your diet as well. Juicing is just part of the weight loss equation. Diet and Exercising are important as well.

Lastly, if you have enjoyed and benefited from this book, please kindly share it with your friends and family so that they too can benefit too. You can easily do take by sharing your thoughts by leaving a review for this book on Amazon.

Thank you and Have an Awesome Week Ahead!

ABOUT THE AUTHOR

Roy Nolan is an avid chef, self-taught nutritionist and wellness enthusiast. His strong passion for healthy living, dieting, nutrition and weight loss leads to his successful transformation. He is an entrepreneur, a fitness buff and a part-time author.

Since childhood, Roy, a young growing boy has a huge appetite, especially during his teenage years. His weight begun to balloon quickly and by the age of 18, he was already 120kg.

Roy hates looking at himself in the mirror. He decided to put an end to it and love himself. Like everyone, he looked for an easy way out and tried almost every type of diet pills to be skinny again. But none of it worked and worst some of the pills induced terrible side effects.

Eventually, Roy realized that this is a vicious cycle and is not a long-term solution. Roy started to learn about the potential benefits of diets such as Paleo, Atkins & Ketogenic and decided that Ketogenic diet could be the answer to his problem.

Today, his successful transformation was made possible with years of research (since 2006) and applying the right actions. Roy decided to compile and share his knowledge of different diets in some of the books he has written.

In his spare time, Roy likes to hit the gym and participate in runs.

Did you like this book?

If you would like to read more great books like this one, why not subscribe to our website and receive **LIFETIME Updates** on all our latest promotions, upcoming books and new book releases, and free books or gifts that we occasionally pamper our loyal members.

https://goo.gl/Zh2xbe

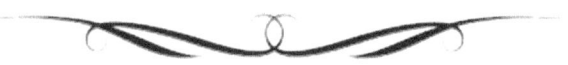

Check out Roy's other proud works below if you didn't get a chance or follow Roy at
https://goo.gl/hU7QZD

Thanks for reading! I hope that you have created new tasty juices for juices for a healthier living. Please add a short review on Amazon Amazon
and let me know what you thought! - Roy

PAVO PRESS

We would like to thank you again for reading this book. Lots of effort, planning and time were committed to ensure that you are receiving the best possible information with as much value as possible. We hope you have unlocked the values from this book.

If you've feel that you have benefited and find that this book is helpful, we would like to ask for a small favor.

Please kindly leave a positive review on Amazon or your favorite social media.

Your review is appreciated and will go a long way to motivate us in producing more quality books for your reading pleasure and needs.

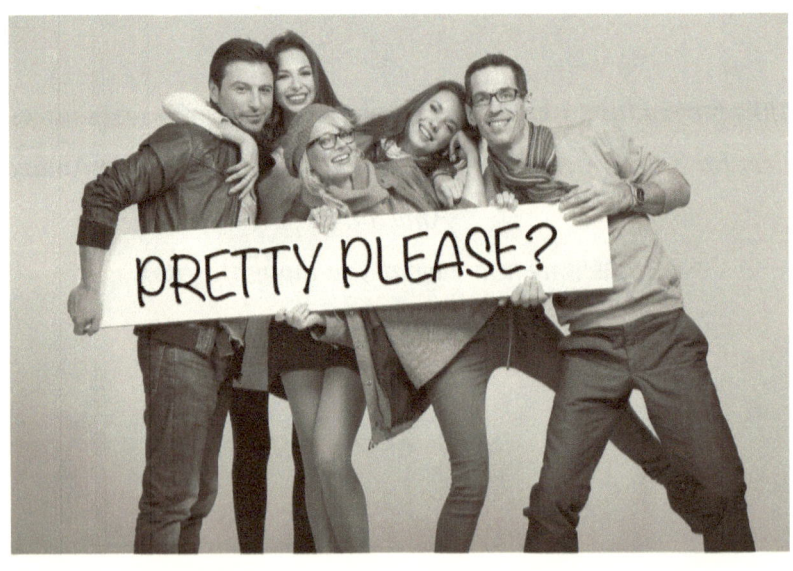